Unleashing Your Purpose

ANNA DE LA TORRE

ISBN: 9798386081140

DEDICATION

This book is dedicated to you.

Because you might not have all the answers but you keep looking for them.

CONTENTS

ACKNOWLEDGMENTS

I could not have undertaken this journey without my princess, my daughter. I learn so much from her every single day. She is the reason of my existence. Words could never describe how magical my baby girl is. I am beyond blessed for having her in my life. To be able to watch her live is the most precious gift I have. To my Princess.

1 UNDERSTANDING FULFILLMENT

Fulfillment is an elusive concept that can be difficult to define. At its core, fulfillment is a deep sense of satisfaction and contentment that arises from living a life that aligns with your values and brings meaning and purpose to your days. It is a state of being that encompasses both joy and peace, and it is something that many people strive for, but not all achieve.

In order to understand what fulfillment means, it is important to consider what it is not. Fulfillment is not the same thing as happiness, which is often fleeting and dependent on external circumstances. Fulfillment is a deeper, more lasting sense of satisfaction that comes from living a life that is meaningful to you. It is not something that can be bought or achieved through external validation, but is instead a state of mind that arises from within.

To begin to uncover your own sense of fulfillment, it can be helpful to examine your values and priorities. What matters most to you in life? What are your core beliefs and principles? What brings you joy and makes you feel alive? These are all important questions to consider when exploring the concept of fulfillment.

Another key component of fulfillment is a sense of purpose. Having a clear sense of direction and a feeling that you are contributing to something larger than yourself can be incredibly fulfilling. This could involve pursuing a career that aligns with your values, volunteering for a cause that you are passionate about, or simply engaging in hobbies and activities that bring you a sense of purpose and fulfillment.

Finally, it is important to remember that fulfillment is a journey, not a destination. It is not something that can be achieved overnight, but rather a process of self-discovery and growth that evolves over time. By staying present in the moment and focusing on your values and priorities, you can begin to cultivate a sense of fulfillment that will sustain you for years to come.

2 UNCOVERING YOUR PURPOSE

One of the biggest challenges in achieving fulfillment is understanding our purpose. It's a question that many of us struggle with, but finding an answer can be life-changing. When we know our purpose, we have a clear direction and meaning in our lives. In this chapter, we'll explore some strategies for uncovering your purpose.

Reflect on Your Passions and Interests: Often, our purpose is tied to what we're most passionate about. Take some time to reflect on what truly excites you. What activities or interests do you find yourself drawn to? What do you love doing, even if it doesn't feel like work? Consider how you can incorporate those passions into your career or personal life.

Identify Your Strengths: We all have unique strengths and talents, and these can be a clue to our purpose. Consider what you're good at and enjoy doing. Think about what others have praised you for in the past. Reflecting on your strengths can help you identify how you can use your abilities to make a positive impact on the world.

Consider Your Values: Our values play a significant role in shaping our purpose. What matters most to you? What do you stand for? Consider how you can align your purpose with your values. When we live in alignment with our values, we feel a sense of integrity and purpose.

Examine Your Life Story: Our life experiences can also provide clues to our purpose. Consider your life story and how it has shaped you. What challenges have you overcome, and what lessons have you learned? Reflecting on your life experiences can help you identify ways in which you can make a positive impact on others.

Experiment: Sometimes, we don't know our purpose until we try new things. Don't be afraid to experiment and try new activities or pursuits. Exploring different options can help you uncover your purpose and find what truly fulfills you.

Remember, discovering your purpose is a journey, not a destination. Be patient and gentle with yourself as you explore and experiment. By reflecting on your passions, strengths, values, life story, and trying new things, you'll be well on your way to uncovering your purpose and creating a fulfilling life.

3 IDENTIFYING YOUR VALUES

Values are the beliefs and principles that guide our decision-making and behavior. They are the foundation upon which we build our lives and the things that matter most to us. When we live in alignment with our values, we feel a sense of fulfillment and purpose.

However, many of us have never taken the time to identify our values. We may have a vague sense of what matters to us, but we haven't articulated those things clearly. When we don't know our values, it's easy to get swept up in the expectations of others or the cultural norms around us. We may find ourselves living a life that doesn't truly reflect who we are or what we care about.

Identifying our values requires some introspection and reflection. It's not always an easy process, but it's one that can be incredibly illuminating and empowering. Here are some steps to help you identify your values:

Reflect on your past experiences: Think about the moments in your life when you felt most alive, fulfilled, or proud. What values were being expressed in those moments? For example, if you felt most alive when you were volunteering for a cause you care about, then your values may include compassion or service.

Consider what you admire in others: Think about the people you admire most in the world. What values do they embody? For example, if you admire someone for their honesty, then honesty may be a value that matters to you.

Reflect on what brings you joy: What activities or experiences bring you the most joy and fulfillment? What values are being expressed in those moments? For example, if spending time in nature brings you joy, then your values may include connection or harmony.

Make a list of your values: Once you've reflected on these questions, make a list of the values that feel most important to you. You may end up with a long list, but try to distill it down to a few key values that feel most essential to who you are.

Prioritize your values: Once you have your list of values, prioritize them in order of importance. This can help you make decisions and choices that are in alignment with your values.

Identifying your values is a powerful first step in creating a life that is fulfilling and meaningful. When you know what matters most to you, you can make choices that are in alignment with your values and live a life that feels authentic and true to who you are.

4 THE IMPORTANCE OF IDENTIFYING YOUR VALUES

Living a fulfilling and meaningful life is closely tied to aligning your actions and decisions with your personal values. Your values represent what is most important to you, and they guide your behaviors, decisions, and relationships. When your actions align with your values, you feel a sense of purpose, fulfillment, and contentment.

However, many people have never taken the time to identify their core values. They may have a vague idea of what they value, but they have never sat down and thought deeply about it. As a result, they may find themselves feeling unfulfilled or like they are living a life that is not truly their own.

Identifying your values is an essential step in uncovering your purpose and creating a life that is fulfilling and meaningful. Here are some reasons why:

Your values guide your decisions: When you have a clear understanding of your values, you can use them to make decisions that align with what is most important to you. This helps you feel confident in your choices and prevents you from feeling like you are compromising on what you truly want.

Your values give you a sense of direction: When you know what you value, you have a clearer sense of what you want to achieve in life. This helps you set goals that are aligned with your values and gives you a sense of purpose and direction.

Your values help you prioritize your time and energy: When you know what you value, you can prioritize your time and energy accordingly. This helps you avoid getting caught up in activities or relationships that do not serve your highest priorities.

Your values give you a sense of identity: Your values are an essential part of who you are, and they can help you feel a sense of identity and belonging. When you live in alignment with your values, you feel more authentic and true to yourself.

So how do you identify your values? Here are some steps you can take:

Reflect on what is most important to you: Take some time to reflect on what is most important to you in life. Think about the things that bring you the most joy, fulfillment, and satisfaction.

Identify your core values: Based on your reflections, identify the core values that are most important to you. These may include things like family, honesty, creativity, or freedom.

Prioritize your values: Once you have identified your core values, prioritize them in order of importance. This can help you make decisions that are aligned with your highest priorities.

Use your values to guide your decisions: As you go about your daily life, use your values to guide your decisions and actions. This will help you live in alignment with what is most important to you and create a life that is fulfilling and meaningful.

Identifying your values is an ongoing process that requires regular reflection and adjustment. As you grow and evolve, your values may also shift and change. However, by taking the time to identify your values and live in alignment with them, you can create a life that is truly fulfilling and meaningful.

5 OVERCOMING OBSTACLES TO FULFILLMENT

Fulfillment is not a destination but a journey, and on this journey, there will be obstacles. Obstacles can take many forms, from external factors such as a lack of resources or unsupportive people, to internal barriers like fear, self-doubt, and limiting beliefs. However, these obstacles do not have to be roadblocks to fulfillment. They can be overcome with the right mindset, strategies, and support.

The first step to overcoming obstacles is to acknowledge and accept them. It's essential to recognize that these obstacles are not a reflection of your worth or abilities but are part of the human experience. Once you accept this fact, you can shift your focus from the obstacle to the solutions.

One of the most effective ways to overcome obstacles is to shift your mindset from a fixed to a growth mindset. A fixed mindset believes that our abilities and intelligence are predetermined and cannot be changed. On the other hand, a growth mindset believes that our abilities and intelligence can be developed and improved through hard work, dedication, and learning. When we have a growth mindset, we are more likely to embrace challenges, persist in the face of setbacks, and see failures as opportunities for growth.

Another strategy for overcoming obstacles is to break them down into smaller, more manageable steps. When we face a large obstacle, it can feel overwhelming and paralyzing. However, when we break it down into smaller tasks, it becomes more manageable and less intimidating. This approach can help us to move forward and make progress, even if it's just one small step at a time.

Another crucial factor in overcoming obstacles is having a support system.

This can be family, friends, colleagues, mentors, or coaches who provide encouragement, guidance, and accountability. It's essential to surround ourselves with people who believe in us, challenge us, and support us on our journey to fulfillment.

Finally, it's important to recognize that obstacles can be opportunities for growth and learning. When we face challenges and overcome them, we become more resilient, adaptable, and confident. We also learn valuable lessons that we can apply to future obstacles and challenges.

In conclusion, obstacles are an inevitable part of the journey to fulfillment. However, they do not have to stop us from achieving our goals and living a meaningful life. By shifting our mindset, breaking down obstacles into smaller steps, building a support system, and seeing obstacles as opportunities for growth, we can overcome any obstacle that comes our way.

6 DEVELOPING A GROWTH MINDSET TO CULTIVATE FULFILLMENT

Fulfillment is not a one-time event; it is a continuous process that requires constant growth and development. In order to live a fulfilling life, it's essential to adopt a growth mindset, which is the belief that our abilities and talents can be developed through hard work, dedication, and perseverance.

A growth mindset enables us to see challenges as opportunities for growth and to view failure as a learning experience rather than a setback. When we have a growth mindset, we believe that we can improve our skills and abilities, and we are more likely to take risks and pursue our goals.

Here are some ways to develop a growth mindset:

Embrace challenges: Instead of avoiding challenges, embrace them as opportunities for growth. Take on tasks that stretch your abilities and push you outside your comfort zone.

Learn from failures: Don't let failure discourage you. Instead, use it as a learning experience to identify areas where you can improve and grow.

Cultivate curiosity: Stay curious about the world around you and actively seek out new experiences and knowledge.

Focus on effort: Instead of focusing on the outcome, focus on the effort you put in. Recognize and celebrate your hard work and progress, even if the outcome isn't what you expected.

Believe in your ability to change: Recognize that you have the power to change and develop your skills and abilities.

Surround yourself with growth-minded individuals: Seek out people who share a growth mindset and can support and encourage you in your growth journey.

Developing a growth mindset is not always easy, and it requires consistent effort and practice. However, it's a powerful tool that can help you cultivate fulfillment and achieve your goals.

When we approach life with a growth mindset, we become more open to new experiences and opportunities, and we are more likely to take on challenges that can lead to personal and professional growth. We are also more likely to view setbacks and failures as opportunities for growth, rather than as roadblocks to our success.

A growth mindset is essential for cultivating fulfillment because it enables us to see the world as a place of endless possibilities and opportunities. With a growth mindset, we can approach our lives with curiosity, passion, and a sense of purpose, which can help us find meaning and fulfillment in all that we do.

In the next chapter, we will explore the importance of developing a sense of purpose and how it can contribute to a fulfilling life.

7 THE IMPORTANCE OF TAKING ACTION

Finding your purpose and aligning with your values is only half of the equation when it comes to living a fulfilling life. The other half is taking action towards your goals and dreams. Without taking action, all the reflection and introspection in the world will not bring about the changes you desire.

Taking action can feel daunting, but it's important to remember that any action, no matter how small, is progress towards your goal. In this chapter, we'll explore why taking action is essential for fulfillment, as well as some strategies for overcoming procrastination and staying motivated.

The Benefits of Taking Action

Taking action towards your goals and dreams has a multitude of benefits, both for your personal growth and for achieving fulfillment in your life. Here are a few reasons why taking action is so important:

Progress: Taking action is the only way to make progress towards your goals. Without action, you are standing still.

Confidence: Taking action builds confidence in yourself and your abilities. Each step you take towards your goal is a reminder that you are capable of making progress.

Momentum: Once you start taking action, it becomes easier to keep going. Momentum builds as you see the results of your efforts.

Learning: Taking action is a valuable learning experience. You will learn from your successes and your failures, and each experience will help you grow and improve.

Overcoming Procrastination

Procrastination is one of the biggest obstacles to taking action towards your goals. It's easy to get caught up in excuses and put things off until later, but this only delays progress and can lead to feelings of guilt and inadequacy.

Here are some strategies for overcoming procrastination:

Break tasks into smaller steps: When a task feels overwhelming, break it down into smaller, more manageable steps. This will make it feel less daunting and easier to get started.

Create a plan: Having a plan of action can help you stay on track and avoid getting sidetracked by distractions. Write down specific steps you will take towards your goal, and when you will take them.

Set deadlines: Deadlines can help create a sense of urgency and motivate you to take action. Set realistic deadlines for each step of your plan.

Get an accountability partner: Having someone to hold you accountable can be a powerful motivator. Find a friend, family member, or coach who will check in with you and help keep you on track.

Staying Motivated

Taking action towards your goals can be challenging, especially when progress feels slow or setbacks occur. Here are some strategies for staying motivated:

Celebrate successes: Celebrating small successes along the way can help keep you motivated and build momentum. Take time to acknowledge your progress and accomplishments.

Visualize your end goal: Visualizing the end result of your efforts can help keep you motivated and focused on the big picture.

Remind yourself of your "why": Remembering why you started on this path can help reignite your motivation and remind you of the importance of your goals.

Take breaks: It's important to take breaks and give yourself time to recharge. Taking a step back can help you come back refreshed and re-energized.

Conclusion

Taking action towards your goals and dreams is an essential part of living a fulfilling life. It may feel daunting at first, but remember that any action, no matter how small, is progress towards your goal. Overcoming procrastination and staying motivated can be challenging, but with the right strategies, you can overcome these obstacles and achieve the fulfillment you desire.

8 EMBRACING FAILURE AND LEARNING FROM IT

Failure is often seen as something negative, but it is important to understand that it is an essential part of growth and success. No one becomes successful without experiencing some degree of failure, and it is through these failures that we can learn and grow.

One of the biggest obstacles to embracing failure is the fear of it. People often fear failure because of the negative emotions that come with it, such as shame, embarrassment, and disappointment. However, it is important to understand that these emotions are natural and temporary, and that they will eventually pass.

The first step in embracing failure is to change your mindset. Failure is not something to be ashamed of, but rather an opportunity to learn and grow. Instead of viewing failure as a negative experience, try to see it as a chance to improve yourself and your circumstances.

Another important aspect of embracing failure is to be resilient. Resilience is the ability to recover from setbacks and continue moving forward. When you experience failure, it is important to take time to reflect on what went wrong and how you can improve in the future. Then, pick yourself up and try again.

It is also important to recognize that failure is not always the result of your actions or lack of effort. Sometimes external factors, such as market conditions or unforeseen circumstances, can lead to failure. In these situations, it is important to not blame yourself, but instead focus on what you can control and how you can adapt to the situation.

Learning from failure is also important in creating a fulfilling and meaningful life. By examining your failures, you can gain valuable insights into what works and what doesn't, and use this knowledge to improve your strategies and approaches in the future.

Finally, it is important to not let failure define you. Your failures do not determine your worth or your potential for success. Instead, focus on your strengths and the progress you have made towards your goals. Celebrate your successes and use them as motivation to continue striving towards your purpose and values.

In conclusion, embracing failure is an important part of achieving fulfillment in life. By changing your mindset, being resilient, recognizing external factors, learning from your failures, and not letting failure define you, you can use failure as a tool for growth and success. Remember, failure is not the end, but rather a stepping stone towards a more fulfilling and meaningful life.

9 FINDING PURPOSE THROUGH SERVICE

We all want to feel that our lives have meaning and purpose. Yet, it can be difficult to find that purpose in our daily lives. Many people find that volunteering or serving others can be a powerful way to find that sense of purpose.

Service can take many forms, from volunteering at a local food bank to donating time to a community organization. The act of giving back to others can be deeply fulfilling, and can help us feel that we are making a positive difference in the world.

One of the key benefits of service is that it can help us gain perspective. When we are focused on our own problems and concerns, it can be easy to lose sight of the bigger picture. Serving others can remind us that we are part of a larger community, and can help us see the struggles that others face.

Service can also help us develop empathy and compassion. When we work with others who are experiencing difficult circumstances, we can gain a better understanding of their challenges and develop a deeper sense of empathy. This can help us become more patient and understanding with those around us, and can lead to stronger, more meaningful relationships.

Another important benefit of service is that it can help us develop new skills and talents. Whether we are volunteering at a local hospital or serving on the board of a community organization, we can gain valuable experience and knowledge that we can use in other areas of our lives.

Finding the right service opportunity can take some time and effort. It's important to choose a cause or organization that resonates with us personally, and that aligns with our values and interests. Some people find that they are most fulfilled when they are working with children, while others may be drawn to environmental causes or social justice issues.

It's also important to be realistic about the time and resources we can commit to service. While it can be tempting to want to do everything we can to help others, it's important to find a balance that allows us to serve effectively without neglecting our own needs and responsibilities.

One of the most powerful ways to find purpose through service is to connect with others who are also passionate about the same cause. Joining a community organization or participating in a service group can be a great way to meet like-minded individuals and build a sense of camaraderie and shared purpose.

Ultimately, finding purpose through service requires us to be open and receptive to the needs of others. It requires us to step outside of our own concerns and focus on the needs of those around us. By doing so, we can find a sense of fulfillment and meaning that can enrich our lives in countless ways.

10 CULTIVATING GRATITUDE AND APPRECIATION

Gratitude is a powerful force that can transform our lives and bring us a sense of joy and fulfillment. It is the practice of recognizing and appreciating the good things in our lives, no matter how small, and acknowledging the efforts of those who have contributed to our well-being.

When we cultivate a mindset of gratitude, we become more aware of the abundance in our lives, and we start to focus on what we have rather than what we lack. This shift in perspective can lead to a happier and more fulfilling life. In this chapter, we will explore the importance of gratitude and ways to cultivate it in our daily lives.

Gratitude is not just a feeling; it is a practice. To cultivate gratitude, we must make it a daily habit. One way to do this is to start a gratitude journal. Each day, write down three things you are grateful for. They can be as simple as having a roof over your head, a warm meal, or a smile from a stranger. By focusing on what you are grateful for, you will start to notice more of the good things in your life.

Another way to cultivate gratitude is to express appreciation to those around you. Take the time to thank your loved ones, friends, and colleagues for their contributions to your life. When you show gratitude, you not only make others feel valued, but you also reinforce your own sense of abundance.

Gratitude can also be cultivated through mindfulness practices. Take a few minutes each day to sit quietly and focus on your breath. As thoughts come and go, simply observe them without judgment. When you find your mind wandering, gently bring your attention back to your breath. This practice of mindfulness can help you become more present in the moment and more aware of the good things in your life.

Another way to cultivate gratitude is to give back to others. When we help others, we not only make a positive impact in their lives, but we also feel a sense of fulfillment and gratitude. Volunteer at a local shelter, donate to a charity, or simply help a neighbor in need. By serving others, you can cultivate a sense of purpose and meaning in your life.

Gratitude is not just a personal practice; it can also be integrated into our relationships and communities. Create a culture of gratitude in your workplace, school, or social group by encouraging others to express appreciation and recognition for each other's contributions. When we acknowledge and celebrate the good things in our lives, we create a positive and supportive environment.

In summary, cultivating gratitude and appreciation can bring immense joy and fulfillment into our lives. By focusing on what we have, expressing appreciation to others, practicing mindfulness, serving others, and creating a culture of gratitude, we can cultivate a sense of abundance and purpose. Start today by writing down three things you are grateful for, and watch as your sense of gratitude and fulfillment grows.

ABOUT THE AUTHOR

Anna De La Torre is an Argentinian writer, a Health and English coach. Who spends her life learning and sharing knowledge to help people overcome their struggles and to achieve a better version of themselves. On her first series of books Own Your Life she encourages people to live their life to the fullest potential.